MCQs in Oral Pathology

MCQs in Oral Pathology

(with Explanatory Answers)

K Karunakaran MDS
Professor
JKK Nataraja Dental College
Kumarapalayam

JAYPEE BROTHERS
MEDICAL PUBLISHERS (P) LTD
New Delhi

Jitendar P Vij
Jaypee Brothers Medical Publishers (P) Ltd
B-3 EMCA House, 23/23B Ansari Road, Daryaganj,
New Delhi 110 002, India Phones: +91-11-23272143, +91-11-23272703,
+91-11-23282021, +91-11-23245672, Rel: 32558559
Fax: +91-11-23276490, +91-11-23245683
e-mail: jaypee@jaypeebrothers.com
Visit our website: www.jaypeebrothers.com

Branches

- 2/B, Akruti Society, Jodhpur Gam Road Satellite
Ahmedabad 380 015, Phones: +91-079-26926233, Rel: +91-079-32988717,
Fax: +91-079-26927094 e-mail: jpamdvd@rediffmail.com
- 202 Batavia Chambers, 8 Kumara Krupa Road Kumara Park East,
Bangalore 560 001, Phones: +91-80-22285971, +91-80-22382956,
Rel: +91-80-32714073, Fax: +91-80-22281761 e-mail: jaypeemedpubbgl@eth.net
- 282 IIIrd Floor, Khaleel Shirazi Estate, Fountain Plaza Pantheon Road,
Chennai 600 008, Phones: +91-44-28193265, +91-44-28194897,
Rel: +91-44-32972089, Fax: +91-44-28193231 e-mail: jpchen@eth.net
- 4-2-1067/1-3, 1st Floor, Balaji Building, Ramkote Cross Road
Hyderabad 500 095, Phones: +91-40-66610020, +91-40-24758498,
Rel:+91-40-32940929, Fax:+91-40-24758499, e-mail: jpmedpub@rediffmail.com
- No. 41/3098, B & B1, Kuruvi Building, St. Vincent Road
Kochi 682 018, Kerala, Phones: 0484-4036109
- 1-A Indian Mirror Street, Wellington Square
Kolkata 700 013, Phones: +91-33-22451926, +91-33-22276404, +91-33-22276415,
Rel: +91-33-32901926, Fax: +91-33-22456075, e-mail: jpbcal@dataone.in
- 106 Amit Industrial Estate, 61 Dr SS Rao Road, Near MGM Hospital, Parel,
Mumbai 400 012, Phones: +91-22-24124863, +91-22-24104532,
Rel: +91-22-32926896, Fax: +91-22-24160828,
e-mail: jpmedpub@bom7.vsnl.net.in
- "KAMALPUSHPA" 38, Reshimbag, Opp. Mohota Science College, Umred Road
Nagpur 440 009 (MS) Phones: Rel: 3245220, Fax: 0712-2704275
e-mail: jaypeenagpur@dataone.in

MCQs in Oral Pathology

First Edition: **2007**

ISBN 81-8061-892-7

Typeset at JPBMP typesetting unit

Printed at Replika Press Pvt. Ltd.

to

My father who was always
inclined towards my prosperity
though he is no more

Preface

MCQs in Oral Pathology is a small attempt to guide the undergraduate dental students to incline towards the basics in oral pathology. I have compiled about 500 questions from all the chapters of Oral Pathology and descriptive answers are given wherever it is necessary.

My sincere thanks to my Principal, Professor K Vijayalakshmi MDS, who made a initial spark for this attempt. I am also grateful to Mrs N Senthamari, secretary JKK Nataraja Dental College, who provided this position to deliver it.

My sincere and heartful thanks to my Professor, TR Saraswathy MDS, MSc (London) who have introduced and mastered me in Oral Pathology.

Also thanks to my mother who stood by my side during my studies. At last but not least I am also grateful to my wife and my son who provided moral support to all my achievements.

K Karunakaran

Contents

Contents

1

Developmental Disturbances of Oral and Paraoral Structures

1. **The following statements regarding clinical character of mandibular micrognathia are true, *except*:**

   A. Severe retrusion of chin
   B. Steep mandibular angle
   C. Severe protrusion of chin
   D. Deficient chin button

   Ans: (C) Mandibular micrognathia means short mandible, results in retrusion of the chin.

2. **The word "Agnathia" denotes:**

   A. Small jaw
   B. Large mandible
   C. Missing maxilla or mandible
   D. Absence of the tongue

   Ans: (C) A=absence Gnathia=jaw

3. **Macrognathia associated with following conditions *except*:**

   A. Pierre Robin syndrome
   B. Paget's disease
   C. Acromegaly
   D. Fibrous dysplasia

   Ans: (A)

4. **The following factors attributed to facial hemihypertrophy *except*:**

   A. Hormonal and chromosomal abnormalities
   B. Incomplete twinning of embryo
   C. Localized alteration of intrauterine development
   D. Iatrogenic abnormolities

   Ans: (D) Iatrogenic produced by doctors during any procedure in the hospital.

5. Van der Woude's syndrome is:

A. Association of pits in the lower lip and cleft lip or cleft palate
B. Double lip and cleft palate
C. Cheilitis granulomatosa, facial paralysis and scrotal tongue
D. None of the above

Ans:(A), Choice (C) Symptom complex of Melkersson-Rosenthal syndrome.

6. Development lip anomaly which resembles Cupid's bow in:

A. Cleft lip
B. Cheilitis granulomatosa
C. Double lip
D. Lip pit

Ans: (C)

7. Superficial suppurative type of cheilitis glandularis also known as:

A. Baelz's disease
B. Cheilitis glandularis apostematosa
C. Myxadenitis labialis
D. None of the above

Ans: (A) Choice "B & C" are other name for deep suppurative disease.

8. Familial generalised intestinal polyposis and pigmented spots on the face, oral cavity and some times hands and feet, are feature of:

A. Peutz-Jeghers syndrome
B. Miescher' syndrome
C. Gardner's syndrome
D. Addison's disease

Ans: (A)

9. Bilateral symmetrical, granular yellow plaque in the buccal mucosa known as:

A. Heck's disease
B. Fordyce's granules
C. Pigmentary disturbances associated with pharmaceutical and other chemicals
D. Benign and malignant pigmented neoplasm.

Ans: (B) Ectopic sebaceous gland in oral cavity is known as Fordyce's granules.

10. Dense diffuse, smooth or nodular growth of the gingival, usually appears the time of eruption of permanent incisor in one or both the arches known as:

A. Hereditary gingival fibromatosis
B. Dilantin gingival hyperplasia
C. Inflammatory gingival hyperplasia
D. Eosinophilic granuloma

Ans: (A) Also called elephantiasis gingiva.

11. Secondary macroglossia occurs in following pathological conditions, *except:*

A. Hyperpituitarism
B. Cretinism
C. Tumour of the tongue
D. Congenital

Ans: (D) Primary macroglossia occurs in congenital condition.

12. Partial cleft in the tongue results due to:

A. Incomplete merging and failure of groove oblitration by underlying mesenchyme
B. Failure of fusion lateral lingual swelling
C. Failure of fusion of occipital myotomes
D. All of the above

Ans: (A)

13. Ovoid or rhomphoid shaped reddish patch on dorsal surface of the tongue is a feature of:

A. Benign migratory glossitis
B. Median rhomboid glossitis
C. Hairy tongue
D. Lingual tonsil

Ans: (B) Results due to failure of fusion of tuberculum impar with two lateral swelling.

14. Hypertrophic filliform papillae a histopathologic feature of:

A. Geographic tongue
B. Hairy tongue
C. Central papillary atrophy of the tongue
D. Wandering rash

Ans: (B) Hypertrophic filliform papilla, secondary pigmentation gives black hairy tongue appearance clinically.

15. Following statements are true about varix, *except*:

A. Dilated tortuous vein
B. Increased hydrostatic pressure in the venous end and poorly supported by surrounding tissue
C. Due to depapillation of ventral surface of the tongue
D. Common in ranine veins

Ans: (C)

16. Kimura's disease is:

A. Angiolymphoid hyperplasia with eosinophilia
B. Angiolymphoid follicular lymph node malformation
C. Reactive lymphoid hyperplasia
D. All of the above

Ans: (A) Atypical endothelial proliferation, lymphoid aggregates numerous eosinophils and chronic inflammatory cell infiltration.

17. The term xerostomia denotes:

A. Dryness of the eye
B. Dryness of the stomach
C. Dryness of the mouth
D. Increased salivation

Ans: (C)

18. The following factors are causes for xerostomia, *except*:

A. Radiation therapy
B. Bell's palsy
C. Administration of atropine and antihistaminic drugs
D. Vitamin A deficiency

Ans: (B) Drooping of saliva seen in Bell's palsy.

19. The term "Atresia" denotes:

A. Congenital occlusion or absence of one or more of the major salivary gland ducts
B. Widespread distribution of normal accessory salivary glands
C. Hyperplasia of the palatal glands
D. Atrophy of the salivary glands

Ans: (A)

20. True generalized microdontia commonly occurs in:

A. Hereditary ectodermal dysplasia
B. Pituitary dwarfism
C. Congenital syphilis
D. Down's syndrome

Ans: (B)

21. The following statements are true regarding Stafne's cyst *except*:

A. It's developmental lingual mandibular salivary gland depression
B. It's a type of salivary gland aberrancy
C. Generally located between mandibular canal and inferior border of the mandible
D. It lies above the mandibular canal

Ans: (D)

22. True generalized macrodontia is associated with:

A. Pituitary gigantism B. Hemihypertrophy of the face
C. Hyperthyroidism D. Trisomy 21

Ans : (A)

23. All are true about gemination *except*:

A. Anomaly results due to division of single tooth germ by an invagination
B. Union of two normaly separated tooth germs
C. Two completely or incompletely separated crowns that have a single root and root canal
D. Difficult to differentiate between gemination and a case in which there has been fusion between a normal tooth and a supernumerary tooth

Ans: (B)

24. An angulation or a sharp bend or curve in the root or crown of a formed tooth known as:

A. Dens in dente
B. Dilated composite odontome
C. Dilaceration
D. Taurodontism

Ans: (C)

25. The following statements are true about Talon's cusp *except*:

A. Present in the lingual aspect of maxillary posteriors
B. Projects lingually from the cingulum areas of a maxillary or mandibular permanent incisor
C. One of the symptom in Rubinstein-Taybi syndrome
D. Composed of normal enamel dentin and pulp

Ans: (A)

26. The tooth most commonly affected in condition called 'Dens in Dente' is:

A. Maxillary canine
B. Maxillary lateral incisor
C. Mandibular central incisor
D. All of the above

Ans: (B)

27. An accessory cusp or globule of enamel on the occlusal surface between buccal and lingual cusps of premolar is called:

A. Dens evaginatus
B. Dens invaginatus
C. Talon's cusp
D. Enameloma

Ans: (A) Dens evaginatus occurs due to proliferation and evagination of enamel organ along with dental papilla during development.

28. "Bull like Teeth" seen in which developmental anomaly:

A. Mesiodens
B. Taurodontism
C. Dens invaginatus
D. Talon's cusp

Ans: (B) In Taurodontism the teeth appear similar to cud chewing animals.

29. True anodontia (missing all the teeth) is frequently associated with:

A. Hereditary ectodermal dysplasia
B. Chondroectodermal dysplasia
C. Hereditary amelogenesis imperfecta
D. Osteogenesis imperfecta

Ans: (A) Absence of teeth, sweat glands, and sebaceous gland.

30. Most frequently congenitally missing teeth in human dentition are:

A. Third molars
B. Lateral incisors
C. Maxillary canine
D. Mandibular premolars

Ans: (A)

31. The term " Mesiodens" denotes:

A. Supernumerary tooth situated between maxillary central incisors
B. Supernumerary tooth situated mesial to the 3rd molar
C. Supernumerary tooth mesial to the mandibular lateral incisor
D. Supernumerary tooth around the maxillary premolar

Ans: (A)

32. Following symptoms are features of Gardner's syndrome, *except:*

A. Multiple polyposis of the large intestine
B. Epidermial or sebaceous cyst, and osteoma of the bone
C. Desmoid tumours and multiple supernumerary teeth
D. Skin pigmentations

Ans: (D)

33. "Amelogenesis imperfecta" occurs due to the disturbance of:

A. Ectoderm
B. Ectomesenchyme
C. Mesoderm
D. Endoderm

Ans: (a) Enamel derived from ectoderm

34. Histopathological feature of hypomaturative amelogenesis imperfecta is:

A. Absence enamel matrix
B. Defects of matrix structure
C. Alteration in enamel rod and rod sheath
D. No alteration in histology of enamel

Ans: (C)

35. All are true about environmental enamel hypoplasia, *except:*

A. Both deciduous and permanent dention are affected
B. Only enamel is affected
C. Both enamel and dentin are affected
D. It is caused by environmental factors

Ans: (B)

36. Turner's hypoplasia is:

A. Enamel hypoplasia due to local infection or trauma
B. Enamel hypoplasia due to congenital syphilis
C. Enamel hypoplasia due to birth injuries
D. Enamel hypoplasia due to hypocalcemia

Ans: (A) Unusual type of hypoplasia affecting a single tooth, most commonly maxillary central incisor, involved tooth is called " Turner's tooth".

37. Characteristic "screw- driver' shaped central incisor seen in congenital syphilis, these teeth are termed as:

A. "Hutchinson's teeth" B. Mulberry teeth
C. Moon's molar D. Fournier's molars

Ans. (A) All other choices referred to congenital syphilitic molars.

38. Mottled enamel is due to:

A. Fluorosis B. Hypocalcemia
C. Exanthematous fever D. Amelogenesis imperfecta

Ans: (A)

39. Following statements are true, regarding Type II dentinogenesis imperfecta, *except:*

A. Most frequently referred to as hereditary opalescent dentin
B. It is inherited as an autosomal dominant trait
C. Both deciduous and permanent teeth equally affected
D. It is also called " Brandywine type"

Ans: (D) It's Type III dentinogenesis imperfecta.

40. " Shell teeth" is a roentgenographic feature of:

A. Type III dentinogenesis imperfecta
B. Type II dentinogenesis imperfecta
C. Both type I and III
D. Both Type I and II.

Ans: (A)

41. " Rootless teeth" term denotes:

A. Dentinogenesis imperfecta
B. Regional dentin dysplasia
C. Dentin dysplasia
D. Odontogenesis imperfecta

Ans: (C)

42. "Lava flowing around boulders" is a histological characteristic of:

A. Dentin dysplasia Type I
B. Dentin dysplasia Type II
C. Dentinogenesis imperfecta Type I
D. Type III dentinogenesis imperfecta

Ans: (A)

43. "Ghost teeth" characteristic roentgenographic feature of:

A. Dentin dysplasia
B. Regional odontodysplasia
C. Dentinogenesis imperfecta
D. Osteogenesis imperfecta

Ans: (B) Both enamel and dentin appear very thin, results in radiodensity gives ghost appearance.

44. Deciduous teeth that have erupted at birth are called:

A. Natal teeth
B. Neonatal teeth
C. Supernumerary teeth
D. Pink tooth

Ans: (A) Prematurely erupting in first 30 days of life is called neonatal teeth.

45. Fissural cyst formed in between medial nasal process and the maxillary process is called:

A. Median palatal cyst
B. Globulomaxillary cyst
C. Median anterior maxillary cyst
D. Incisive canal cyst

Ans: (B) Usually between maxillary lateral incisor and canine.

2

Disease of Pulp and Periapical Tissues

1. Prime cause for pulpitis is:

A. Dental caries
B. Fracture of the tooth
C. Trauma
D. Chemical irritation due to restorative materials

Ans: (A)

2. Pulpitis due to bacteremia, known as:

A. Aerodontalgia
B. Seadiver's pulpitis
C. Anacorotic pulpitis
D. Granulomatous pulpitis

Ans: (C)

3. "Pulpitis clausa" refers:

A. Open pulpitis
B. Closed pulpitis
C. Focal reversible pulpitis
D. Acute pulpitis

Ans: (B)

4. The term "Sub total pulpitis" denotes:

A. Diseased pulp confined to pulp chamber
B. Diseased pulp confined to pulp chamber and pulp horn
C. Diseased pulp confined to root canal
D. Entire pulp under inflammation

Ans: (B)

5. " Lancinating" type of pain is a characteristic feature of:

A. Focal reversible pulpitis
B. Chronic pulpitis
C. Pulp polyp
D. Acute pulpitis

Ans: (D)

6. **"Pulp polyp" also known as:**
   A. Chronic hyperplastic pulpitis
   B. Acute reversible pulpitis
   C. Pulp hyperemia
   D. Pink tooth

   Ans: (A)

7. **Intensity of pain increased when patient lies down, is a characteristic feature of:**
   A. Acute reversible pulpitis
   B. Acute pulpitis
   C. Chronic pulpitis
   D. Chronic hyperplastic pulpitis

   Ans: (B)

8. **Teeth most commonly involved by pulp polyp are:**
   A. 3rd molar
   B. 2nd molar and deciduous molar
   C. Deciduous molar and 1st permanent molar
   D. Incisors

   Ans: (C) These teeth have excellent blood supply and high tissue resistance in young age.

9. **Possibility of epithelial implantation in pulp polyp are, *except:***
   A. Gingival epithelium
   B. Buccal mucosa
   C. Shedded epithelium from oral mucosa
   D. Respiratory epithelium

   Ans: (D)

10. **First change in roentgenographic features of periapical lesions are:**
    A. Thickening of periodontal ligament at the root apex results in periapical radiolucency
    B. Bone resorption
    C. Root resorption
    D. Increased radiopaqueness around the periphery of the root

    Ans: (A)

11. In slow growing lesion presence of thin radiopaque line surrounding radiolucent lesion indicates:

A. Reversal line formation
B. Sclerotic bone formation
C. Resting line formation
D. All of the above

Ans: (B) Peripherally outlines the lesion, indicates slowly progressive lesion that has not undergone an acute exacerbation.

12. Foam cells are:

A. Lipid laden macrophages
B. Plasma cells
C. Osteoclasts
D. Mast cells

Ans: (A)

13. Following are possibilities of epithelium in the periapical granuloma, *except:*

A. Epithelial rests of Malassez
B. Respiratory epithelium of the maxillary sinus
C. Oral epithelium either through fistulous tract or from periodontal ligament
D. Odontogenic epithelium from the developing tooth bud

Ans: (D)

14. Dead bone in osteomyelitis are named as:

A. Involucrum
B. Sequestrum
C. Marble bone
D. Dysblastic bone

Ans: (B) Choice A, new bone formation around sequestrated bone.

15. Chronic focal sclerosing osteomyelitis clinically and radiographically always give a diagnostic problem with:

A. Ossifying fibroma
B. Cementyfying fibroma
C. Benign cementoblastoma
D. Ameloblastoma

Ans: (C)

16. Garre's osteomyelitis is also called as:

A. Chronic diffuse osteomyelitis
B. Chronic focal osteomyelitis
C. Chronic osteomyelitis with proliferative periostitis
D. Florid osseous dysplasia

Ans: (C)

17. Dental abscess usually caused by:

A. Staphylococcus
B. Streptococcus
C. Pneumococcus
D. Gonococcus

Ans: (A)

18. Cellulitis is usually associated with Streptococcus, because:

A. It is a common organism causing dental caries
B. It releases hyaluronidase, which cleaves intercellular substances
C. Streptococcus never causes cellulitis
D. Both A and B are correct

Ans: (B)

19. Ludwig's angina is a severe cellulitis involving:

A. Bilateral sub-mandibular, sub-lingual, sub-mental
B. Unilateral sub-mandibular, sub-lingual and sub-mental
C. Sub-lingual and sub-mental
D. Bilateral sub-mandibular

Ans: (A)

20. Death due to Ludwig's angina primary because of:

A. Severe bacteremia
B. Septicemia
C. Edema of the glottis causing suffocation
D. All of the above

Ans: (C)

21. Common route of spread of infection from oral and para-oral structures to cavernous sinus is:

A. External jugular vein B. Internal jugular vein
C. Angular vein D. Pterygoid plexus of vein

Ans: (D)

22. Board-like swelling in the floor of the mouth, elevation of the tongue is a feature of:

A. Cavernous sinus thrombosis
B. Ludwig's angina
C. Submandibular abscess
D. Infection in the floor of the mouth

Ans: (B)

23. Exophthalmos, paralysis of the extraocular muscles, impairment of vision is a clinical feature of:

A. Maxillary sinusitis
B. Ludwig's angina
C. Cavernous sinus thrombosis
D. Meningeal infection

Ans: (C)

24. Discharge of pus into the nose, fetid odour, fever, malaise, pain over maxilla on palpation, referral pain over teeth, sometimes ear are feature of:

A. Acute maxillary sinusitis
B. Chronic maxillary sinusitis
C. Periapical infection in maxillary first molar
D. Infratemporal space infection

Ans: (A)

25. Microorganism or its toxic substances metastasis to distant site are known as:

A. Focus of infection B. Focal infection
C. Metastatic infection D. All of the above

Ans: (B)

3

Dental Caries

1. **Dental caries is a:**
   A. Contagious disease
   B. Microbial disease
   C. Inflammatory disease
   D. Autoimmune disease

   Ans: (B)

2. **Primary destruction in process of dental caries is characterized by:**
   A. Demineralisation of inorganic substances
   B. Destruction of organic substances
   C. Both the process occurs simultaneously
   D. None of the above

   Ans: (A)

3. **What is true about clinical manifestation of dental caries:**
   A. Persist throughout life even after the treatment
   B. Completely cured after restoration
   C. Controlled after antibiotic therapy
   D. Totally arrested after fluoridation

   Ans: (A)

4. **Clinical finding of dental caries in brachycephalic man of the neolithic period are:**
   A. Cervical areas were more frequent site
   B. Occlusal area were commonly affected
   C. Root caries
   D. Proximal caries

   Ans: (A)

5. Organisms responsible for dental caries are:

A. *Staphylococcus*
B. *Streptococcus mutans*
C. *Streptococcus mitis*
D. *Streptococcus sanguis*

Ans: (B)

6. Primitive, raw foods, influence on dental caries:

A. Increase the incidence of dental caries
B. Decrease the incidence of dental caries
C. No influence on dental caries
D. Similar effect as modern diet

Ans: (B) Unrefined, roughaged diet cleanses the teeth of adherent depris during masticatory excursions.

7. Following types are categorized under Pit and Fissure caries, *except:*

A. Occlusal surface of molars and premolars
B. Buccal and lingual surface of molars
C. Lingual surface of the maxillary incisors
D. Cervical areas of all the teeth

Ans: (D) It is type of smooth surface caries.

8. Caries that occurs in immediate vicinity of a restoration is known as:

A. Chronic dental caries
B. Arrested caries
C. Recurrent caries
D. Nursing bottle caries

Ans: (C) It occurs due to improper marginal adaptation.

9. " Eburnated dentin" seen in:

A. Recurrent caries
B. Acute caries
C. Nursing bottle caries
D. Arrested caries

Ans: (D) It appears brownish, polished, shiny on surface.

10. Statement regarding nursing bottle caries are true, *except:*

A. Carious destruction affects four maxillary incisor teeth
B. Mandibular incisors not affected by nursing bottle caries
C. It is a type of acute dental caries and affects severely
D. It is a type of recurrent caries

Ans: (D)

11. Clinical character of arrested caries are follows, *except:*

A. Presence of brown pigmentation
B. Change from soft to hard texture
C. No progress in size of the lesion
D. Progress of lesion immaterial to the pigmentation

Ans: (D) Progress of lesion can be detected by loss of pigmentation.

12. Commonly used chemicals to arrest the dental caries is:

A. Stannous fluoride 22 to 25%
B. Stannous fluoride 10 %
C. Tetracycline topical solution
D. Chlorhexidine topical application

Ans: (A)

13. The earliest manifestation of dental caries in enamel are:

A. Brown discolouration
B. Smooth chalky white area
C. Black discolouration
D. Loss of surface luster and roughness

Ans: (B)

14. First histopathological change in enamel caries is:

A. Loss of interprismatic substances and prominence of enamel rods
B. Roughening of enamel rods
C. Appearance of transverse striations in the enamel rods
D. Accentuation of incremental lines of retzius

Ans: (A and B)

15. In pyramidal shaped pit and fissure caries, base of the pyramid is towards the:

A. Surface of the tooth
B. Dentinoenamel junction
C. Mesial side
D. Distal side

Ans: (B)

16. Microorganisms found in the dentinal tubules, before the clinical evidence of dental caries are termed:

A. Primary bacteria
B. Pioneer bacteria
C. Acidogenic bacteria
D. Proteolytic bacteria

Ans: (B)

17. Histopathological feature of early dentinal changes in dental caries is:

A. Sclerotic dentin formation
B. Transparent dentin formation
C. Dead tracts
D. Fatty degeneration of Tome's fibers

Ans: (D)

18. The tooth which contains more amount of globular dentin is termed:

A. Malacotic or soft tooth B. Pink tooth
C. Tome's tooth D. Carious prone tooth

Ans: (A)

19. These are the four destructive lesion commonly found in the root, *except:*

A. Abrasion and erosion
B. Idiopathic resorption
C. Caries
D. Fracture

Ans: (D)

20. Best view of X-ray advised for diagnosing proximal caries is:

A. Bite wing X-ray
B. Occlusal view
C. Intraoral periapical view
D. OPG X-rays

Ans: (A)

21. Following statements are true regarding mechanism of action of ingested fluoride *except*:

A. Alteration of structure of the developing tooth

B. Inhibits enzymes by inactivating the co-enzyme portion of the enolase system

C. Fluoride has bacterisidal action, which prevents acidogenic bacteria

D. Prevents corbohydrate degradation

Ans: (C)

22. Following measures are controlling dental caries mechanically *except:*

A. Prophylaxis by dentist

B. Incorporation of detergent foods in the diet

C. Mouth rinsing

D. Water fluoridation

Ans: (D) Its chemical measure to control dental caries.

23. Most accepted theory regarding etiology of dental caries is:

A. Proteolytic theory
B. Proteolytic chelation theory
C. Acidogenic theory
D. Chemicoparasitic theory

Ans: (C)

24. Acidogenic theory is proposed by:

A. Cueto and Buonocore (1967)

B. WD Miller (1882)

C. Bunting (1927)

D. Leber and Rotenstin (1867)

Ans: (B)

25. Bacteria responsible for root caries are:

A. Actinomyces species
B. Lactobacilli
C. Streptococcus mutans
D. Veillonella

Ans: (A)

4

Cysts and Tumors of Odontogenic Origin

1. Following cysts are odontogenic origin, *except:*

A. Gingival cyst
B. Eruption cyst
C. Primordial cyst
D. Globulo-maxillary cyst

Ans: (D) It's a fissural cyst.

2. The epithelium associated with odontogenic cysts are follows, *except:*

A. Reduced enamel epithelium of the tooth crown
B. Tooth primordium
C. Glandular epithelium
D. Basal layer of oral epithelium

Ans: (C)

3. Pathogenesis of primordial cyst is:

A. Reduced enamel epithelium
B. Cell rests of Malassez
C. Stellate reticulum of enamel organ prior to enamel formation
D. Basal layer of oral epithelium

Ans: (C)

4. Cystic fluid accumulation between the reduced enamel epithelium and tooth crown, occurs in:

A. Dentigerous cyst
B. Gingival cyst
C. Apical periodontal cyst
D. Lateral periodontal cyst

Ans: (A)

5. **Very common complication of dentigerous cyst is:**
   A. Pathological fracture
   B. Ameloblastoma
   C. Mucoepidermoid carcinoma
   D. Epidermoid carcinoma

   Ans: (B)

6. **Following features are Vickers and Gorlin criteria for potentiality of dentigerous cyst becoming a ameloblastoma, *except:***
   A. Hyperchromatism of basal cell nuclei
   B. Palisading with polarization of basal cells
   C. Vacuolization with intercellular spacing of the lining epithelium.
   D. Sprouting or budding and protruding of epithelial island from lining epithelium

   Ans: (D)

7. **Most common etiology for radicular cyst is:**
   A. Dental caries B. Trauma
   C. Periodontitis D. Both A and B

   Ans: (D)

8. **Bohn's nodule or Epstein's pearl filled with:**
   A. Keratin B. Mucus
   C. Collagen D. None of the above

   Ans: (A) These are found in the midpalatine raphe.

9. **Following features are histopathology of odontogenic keratocyst *except:***
   A. Corrugated parakeratinized surface layer
   B. 6 to 10 layers of palisaded columnar basal layer
   C. Presence of sattelite cyst
   D. Presence of mucus cells in the lining epithelium

   Ans: (D) Presence of mucus cells is a h/p feature of dentigerous cyst.

10. Following statements are true regarding recurrence of Odontogenic Keratocyst *except:*

A. Presence of daughter cyst
B. Detachment of epithelium and connective tissue, complete enucleation is usually not possible
C. Cyst wall is thin and friable
D. Increased mitotic activity

Ans: (D)

11. Multiple odontogenic keratocyst, mandibular prognathism, cutaneous and ophthalmic anomalies are feature of:

A. Basal cell nevus syndrome
B. Gardner's syndrome
C. Still's disease
D. Craniomandibular dysostosis

Ans: (A)

12. Following tumors are odontogenic ectodermal tumors *except:*

A. Ameloblastoma
B. Calcifying epithelial odontogenic tumor
C. Cementoblastoma
D. Adenomatoid odontogenic tumor

Ans: (C) It's a odontogenic mesenchymal tumor.

13. Most commonly occurring odontogenic tumors are:

A. Ameloblastoma
B. Cementoblastoma
C. CEOT
D. AOT

Ans: (A)

14. Histological transformation of odontogenic epithelium with a malignant feature is called:

A. Ameloblastoma
B. Ameloblastic carcinoma
C. Malignant ameloblastoma
D. Primary intra-alveolar carcinoma

Ans: (B)

15. Discrete island of odontogenic epithelium, composed peripheral layer of columnar cells, central polygonal cells, are histopathological feature of:

A. Plexiform type of ameloblastoma
B. AOT
C. Unicystic ameloblastoma
D. Follicular type of ameloblastoma

Ans: (D)

16. In granular type ameloblastoma granular appearance is due to:

A. Lysosomes B. Mitochondria
C. Golgi apparatus D. Rough endoblastic reticulum

Ans: (A) Granular appearance represents lysosomal aggregates.

17. Pindborg's tumor is also called as:

A. Adeno-ameloblastoma
B. Adamantinoma
C. Calcifying epithelial odontogenic tumor
D. Squamous odontogenic tumor

Ans: (C)

18. "Driven Snow" appearance in roentgenographic feature of:

A. CEOT
B. Odontome
C. Ameloblastic odontoma
D. Calcifying epithelial odontogenic cyst

Ans: (A) Scattered fleck of calcification throughout the radiolucency gives driven snow appearance radiographically.

19. 'Liesegang ring' type of calcification is a characteristic feature of:

A. CEOC B. CEOT
C. Ameloblastic fibro-odontoma D. Odontoma

Ans: (B)

20. Histopathologically amyloid deposition is a feature of:

A. Ameloblastoma
B. Adeno-ameloblastoma
C. CEOT
D. Both B and C

Ans: (D)

21. Following lesions are hamartomas, *except:*

A. Hemangioma
B. Odontoma
C. AOT
D. Ossifying fibroma

Ans: (D)

22. Hamartamatous odontogenic lesion composed of dental tissues is called:

A. Benign mixed odontogenic tumor
B. Odontoma
C. Teratoma
D. All of the above

Ans: (B)

23. The calcified dental tissue arranged as a irregular mass not showing morphological similarity even to rudimentary tooth is called:

A. Compound composite odontoma
B. Enameloma
C. Complex composite odontoma
D. Dentinoma

Ans: (C)

24. Ghost cells are seen in:

A. Odontoma
B. CEOT
C. CEOC
D. Both A and C

Ans: (D) These are pale eosinophilic swollen epithelial cells that have lost nucleus but show a faint outline of the cellular and nuclear membrane.

25. **Dark cells, pale cells, large quantities of hyaluronic acid are histopathologic feature of:**
    A. Odontogenic myxoma
    B. Central odontogenic fibroma
    C. Peripheral odontogenic fibroma
    D. Central odontogenic fibroma (WHO) type

    Ans: (A)

5

Bacterial, Viral and Mycotic Infections

1. **Scarlet fever caused by:**
   A. Beta hemolytic streptococci
   B. Alfa hemolytic streptococci
   C. Staphylococci
   D. Cornybacterium diphtheriae

   Ans: (A) It rcleases erythrogenic toxin, also causes tonsillitis, pharyngitis.

2. **Strawberry tongue "Raspberry tongue," are oral manifestation of:**
   A. Diphtheria B. Tuberculosis
   C. Measles D. Scarlet fever

   Ans: (D) White coating with hyperemic fungiform papillae are called "Strawberry tongue", loss of coating with deep red, smooth, glistening surface of the tongue described as "Raspberry tongue"

3. **Kleb's-Löffler bacillus causes:**
   A. Tuberculosis B. Diphtheria
   C. Leprosy D. Uveoparotid fever

   Ans: (B)

4. **"Scrofula" is *Mycobacterial tuberculous* infection of the:**
   A. Skin
   B. Sub-maxillary and cervical lymph node
   C. Gingiva D. Tongue

   Ans: (B)

5. **Lupus vulgaris is a:**
   A. Primary tuberculous infection of the bone
   B. Pulmonary tuberculosis
   C. Primary tuberculous infection of the skin
   D. Secondary tuberculosis

   Ans: (C)

6. **Caseous necrosis is a positive H/P feature of:**
   A. Sarcoidosis
   B. Tuberculosis
   C. Uvoparotid fever
   D. All of the above

   Ans: (B)

7. **Kveim–Siltzbach test is done for diagnosis of :**
   A. Tuberculosis
   B. Uveoparotid fever
   C. Sarcoidosis
   D. Infectious mononucleosis

   Ans: (C)

8. **Lepra cells are seen in:**
   A. Hansen's disease
   B. Sarcoidosis
   C. Tuberculosis
   D. Actinomycosis

   Ans: (A) It's a vaculated macrophages contains lepra bacilli scattered throughout the lesion.

9. **Actinomycosis is a:**
   A. Mycotic infection
   B. Anaerobic filamentous bacterial infection
   C. Viral infection
   D. Granulomatous disease

   Ans: (B)

10. **Suppurative material cotaining sulfur granules are seen in:**
    A. Tubercular abscess
    B. Leprosy
    C. Actinomycosis
    D. Sarcoidosis

    Ans: (C) These granules are nothing but a actinomycies colonies appears as tiny yellow grains.

11. Following are clinical forms of actinomycosis , *except:*

A. Cervicofacial
B. Abdominal
C. Pulmonary
D. Cardiovascular

Ans: (D)

12. Lues are caused by:

A. *Treponema pallidum*
B. Pseudomonas pseudomallei
C. *Clostridium tetani*
D. Pasteurella tularensis

Ans: (A) Lues or syphilis caused by spirochetes.

13. " Mucous patches" occurs in which stage of syphilis:

A. Primary syphilis
B. Congenital syphilis
C. Tertiary syphilis
D. Secondary syphilis

Ans: (D) Multiple grayish white plaques covering the ulcerated surface, contains numerous spirochetes, highly infective.

14. Tertiary lesion, frequently involves skin and mucous membrane is called:

A. Chancre
B. Luetic glossitis
C. Gummatous lesion
D. Mucous patches

Ans: (C)

15. Following lesions are congenital syphilitic manifestations *except:*

A. Irregular thickening of the sternoclavicular portion of the clavicle
B. Hutchinson's triad
C. High palatal arch
D. Aortic aneurysm

Ans: (D) It's a tertiary syphilitic cardiovascular manifestation.

16. Rapidly spreading soft tissue gangrene of the oral and facial tissues are called:

A. Pyogenic granuloma
B. Noma
C. Anug
D. Herpes simplex infection

Ans: (B) Also called cancrum oris or gangrenous stomatitis occurs in debilitated or nutritionally deficient persons.

17. Herpes simplex type I usually causes lesions in:

A. Lower body skin
B. Genital region
C. Face, lips and oral cavity
D. Throughout the body

Ans: (C) Lower body skin and genital region caused by HSV type II virus.

18. Herpes virus is a:

A. DNA virus
B. RNA virus
C. Mixed virus
D. None of the above

Ans: (A)

19. Following viruses are DNA virus *except:*

A. Epstein-Barr virus
B. Cytomegalovirus
C. Human immunodeficiency virus
D. Poxvirus

Ans: (C)

20. Following statement regarding HSV I are true *except:*

A. HSV I could be isolated from primary site of infection about 2 to 6 days
B. HSV I does not remain latent in the site of original infection
C. HSV I could be isolated from the site of infection upto 14 days
D. HSV I remain latent in the trigeminal ganglia.

Ans: (C) It is true for HSV II.

21. Lipschütz's bodies are found in:

A. HSV infection
B. Aphthous ulcer
C. Herpangina
D. Behcet's syndrome

Ans: (A) Intranuclear inclusion bodies, characterized by eosinophilic, ovoid, homogenous structure tend to displace the nucleolus and nuclear material peripherally.

22. Koplic's spots is a oral manifestation of:

A. Smallpox
B. Chikenpox
C. German measles
D. Rubeola

Ans: (D) These are characteristic spots, occurs in the buccal mucosa, bluish-white flecks surrounded by a bright red margin seen in Measles.

23. Herpetic infection of the fingers and hands are known as:

A. Koilonychia
B. Herpetic whitlow
C. Herpetic paranychia
D. None of the above

Ans: (B)

24. These are most common sites for recurrent herpetic Intra-oral lesions *except:*

A. Buccal mucosa
B. Hard palate
C. Attached gingival
D. Alveolar ridge

Ans: (A) Normally never occurs on mobile mucosa.

25. Herpangina is caused by:

A. HSV I
B. HSV II
C. Coxsackie group A virus
D. Poxvirus

Ans: (C)

26. Oral and genital ulceration, ocular lesions, and skin lesion is feature of:

A. Reiter's syndrome
B. Behcet's syndrome
C. Herpangina
D. Recurrent aphthous stomatitis

Ans: (B) It's autoimmune disease, oral ulcers resembles the recurrent aphthous ulcer.

27. **Henderson-Paterson inclusion bodies are present in:**
   A. Molluscum ontagiosum
   B. Condyloma acuminatum
   C. Behcet's syndrome
   D. Reiter's syndrome

   Ans: (A) Intracytoplasmic, eosinophilic inclusion bodies also called molluscum bodies.

28. **Intranuclear and cytoplasmic inclusions in the cells of the salivary gland is a feature of:**
   A. Cytomegalic inclusion disease
   B. Poliomyelitis
   C. Herpangina
   D. Herpes zoster

   Ans: (A)

29. **Organ which is getting affected by mumps is:**
   A. Lungs
   B. Maxillary sinus
   C. Salivary gland
   D. Kidney

   Ans:(C) Parotid gland commonly getting affected by mumps.

30. **Fever, malaise, pain along the course of the involved sensory nerve, linear papular or vesicular eruption of the skin. Clinical features of:**
   A. Cat scratch disease
   B. Herpes zoster
   C. Measles
   D. Foot and mouth disease

   Ans: (B)

31. **Facial paralysis, pain in the external auditory meatus and pinna of the ear vesicular eruption in the oral mucosa, and oro-pharynx are the clinical manifestation of:**
   A. James Ramsay Hunt's syndrome
   B. Infantile paralysis
   C. Herpes zoster
   D. Herpes simplex infection

   Ans: (A) A special form of Herpes zoster infection of the geniculate ganglion, Involvement of external ear and oral mucosa.

32. Mycology the term denotes:

A. Study of infection from the birds
B. Study of fungal infection
C. Both of the above
D. None of the above

Ans: (B)

33. Most common fungal infection of the oral cavity is:

A. Geotrichosis
B. Moniliasis
C. Mucormycosis
D. Cryptococcosis

Ans: (B) Also called candidiasis or thrush.

34. Most suitable media for culture the fungus are:

A. Sabouraud's broth
B. Nystatin
C. Saline broth
D. Lobstein medium

Ans: (A)

35. Commonest candidial species causing oral candidiasis are:

A. *Candida tropicalis*
B. *Candida krusei*
C. *Candida albicans*
D. *Candida stellatoidea*

Ans: (C)

36. A form of candidiasis underneath the denture bearing area is:

A. Acute pseudomembranous candidiasis
B. Chronic atrophic candidiasis
C. Chronic mucocutaneous candidiasis
D. Hyperplastic candidiasis

Ans: (B)

37. The organism appears as large, non-septate hyphae with branching at obtuse angle, tissues showing variable amount of necrosis is the histopathologic feature of:

A. Sporotrichosis
B. Geotrichosis
C. Phycomycosis
D. Candidiasis

Ans: (C)

38. In HIV infected patient most commonest form of candidiasis is:

- **A.** Acute pseudomembranous candidiasis
- **B.** Acute atrophic candidiasis
- **C.** Chronic hyperplastic candidiasis
- **D.** Chronic atrophic candidiasis

Ans: (A)

39. Most appropriate stain to elicit yeast colonies in routine H/P studies are:

- **A.** H and E stains
- **B.** Periodic acid schiff
- **C.** Mucicaramine
- **D.** Periodic alkaline schiff

Ans: (B)

40. Hydatid cyst is a:

- **A.** Parasitic infection
- **B.** Fungal infection
- **C.** Non-odontogenic cyst
- **D.** Fissural cyst

Ans: (A)

6

Disease of Nerves and Muscles

1. **Trigeminal neuralgia also called in following names, *except:***

   A. Tic Douloureux
   B. Trifacial neuralgia
   C. Fothergill's disease
   D. Raeder's syndrome

   Ans: (D) It is paratrigeminal syndrome.

2. **Clinical feature of Trigeminal neuralgia are follows *except:***

   A. Unilateral lancinating type of pain
   B. Presence of "Trigger zones"
   C. Flushing and sweating in the involved side of the face
   D. Intermittent episodes of pain

   Ans: (C) It is a feature of auriculotemporal neuralgia.

3. **The term " Glossopyrosis" denotes:**

   A. Burning tongue
   B. Painful tongue
   C. Hypertrophic tongue
   D. Atrophic tongue

   Ans: (A) Painful tongue is called "Glossodynia".

4. **Dysphagia, sore throat, otalgia, glossodynia, headache, orofacial pain along the course of internal and external carotid arteries due to elongation of styloid process is known as:**

   A. Eagle's syndrome
   B. Horner's syndrome
   C. Jaw winking syndrome
   D. Migraine syndrome

   Ans: (A) Also called carotid artery syndrome.

5. **Miosis, Ptosis, Anhidrosis and vasodilatation of the face is a feature of:**

   A. Eagle's syndrome B. Horner's syndrome
   C. Jaw winking syndrome D. Migraine syndrome

   Ans: (B)

6. **Gustatory sweating is a feature of:**

   A. Auriculotemporal nerve syndrome
   B. Glassopharyngeal syndrome
   C. Trigemenial nerve syndrome
   D. Facial nerve syndrome

   Ans: (A) Frey's syndrome, damage to auriculotemporal nerve and subsequent reinnervation of sweat glands by parasympathetic salivary fibers.

7. **Drooping of the corner of the mouth, watering of the eye, inability to close or wink the eye are features of:**

   A. Facial paralysis B. Frey's syndrome
   C. Trotter's syndrome D. Orofacial dyskinesia

   Ans: (A) Also called Bell's palsy due to facial nerve paralysis.

8. **Deafness, tinnitus, and vertigo are feature of:**

   A. Migraine syndrome B. Méniére's syndrome
   C. Temporal arteritis D. Frey's syndrome

   Ans: (B)

9. **Severe pain after injuring or sectioning of peripheral sensory nerve is termed:**

   A. Causalgia B. Orolingual paresthesia
   C. Glossodynia D. Glossopyrosis

   Ans: (A) Injury occurs after any traumatic dental extraction.

10. **Common muscle in orofacial region affected with myositis ossificans are:**

    A. Buccinator B. Masseter
    C. Orbicularis occuli D. Orbicularis oris

    Ans: (B)

7

Benign and Malignant Tumors of the Oral Cavity

1. Benign neoplasm arising from surface epithelium is called:

A. Fibroma B. Papilloma
C. Keratoacanthoma D. Leukoplakia

Ans (B)

2. Self-healing benign lesion of the oral cavity mimicking oral squamous cell carcinoma:

A. Keratoacanthoma B. Squamous papilloma
C. Squamous acanthoma D. Pigmented cellular nevus

Ans: (A) Clinically and histologicaly mimicks oral carcinoma.

3. Among the pigmented cellular nevus the type which commonly undergoes malignant transformation are:

A. Intradermal nevus B. Compound nevus
C. Spindle cell nevus D. Junctional nevus

Ans: (D)

4. "Abtropfung"or " Drooping off" effect of melonocytes is a histological feature of :

A. Compound nevus B. Intradermal nevus
C. Junctional nevus D. Blue nevus

Ans: (C) Melanocyte breaching the basement membrane growing down into the connective tissue.

5. Following are dysplastic features of epithelium, *except:*

A. Acanthosis B. Basillar hyperplasia
C. Abnormal mitosis D. Epithelial pearl formation

Ans: (A) Increased spinous cell layer is called acanthosis. It's a hyperplastic feature.

6. **Presence of all dysplastic feature within the epithelium, but no break in the basement membrane is a feature of:**

   A. Carcinoma *in situ* B. Verrucous carcinoma
   C. Leukoplakia D. Oral submucous fibrosis

   Ans: (A)

7. **Intracellular edema, large pale nuclei, reticular pattern of spinous cell arrangement is a histologic feature of:**

   A. Leukoedema B. Leukoplakia
   C. Erythroplakia D. Hypertrophic candidiasis

   Ans: (A) Abnormality of the buccal mucosa resembles early leukoplakia.

8. **Most common etiology of basal cell carcinoma is:**

   A. Sunlight B. Tobacco
   C. Hereditary D. Chemical

   Ans: (A) Infrared and UV light radiation are most common etiological factor.

9. **Oral submucous fibrosis is a:**

   A. Pre-cancerous lesion B. Pre-cancerous condition
   C. Malignant lesion D. Inflammatory lesion

   Ans: (B)

10. **Severe burning sensation, trismus, xerostomia, blanching of oral mucous membrane are the clinical features of:**

    A. Oral sub-mucous fibrosis
    B. Leukoplakia
    C. Oral squamous cell carcinoma
    D. Erythroplakia

    Ans: (A)

11. **Rodent ulcer is also called as:**

    A. Basal cell carcinoma B. Squamous cell carcinoma
    C. Verrucous carcinoma D. Malignant melanoma

    Ans: (A)

12. In malignant melanoma melanocytes are restricted to epithelium or epidermis this phase of growth is called:

A. Vertical growth phase B. Radial growth phase
C. Horizontal growth phase D. None of the above

Ans: (B)

13. Following lesions contain giant cells *except:*

A. Aneurysmal bone cyst B. Osteoclastoma
C. Paget's disease D. Verruciform xanthoma

Ans: (D) Xanthoma cells are seen in verruciform xanthoma.

14. Sun-ray appearance in radiographs is a characteristic feature of:

A. Lymphoma B. Malignant melanoma
C. Osteosarcoma D. Osteoma

Ans: (C) Irregular trabeculae of new bone radiating outward periphery of the lesion gives sun-ray appearance.

15. Mycosis fungoides is:

A. Cutaneous T cell lymphoma
B. Fungal infection of the oral cavity
C. Primary lymphoma of the bone
D. Both A and B

Ans: (A)

16. "Starry sky" appearance is a histological feature of:

A. Hodgkin's disease B. Non-Hodgkin's disease
C. Burkitt's lymphoma D. Plasmocytoma

Ans: (C) Lesion filled with darkly stained lymphoreticular cells, with macrophages gives starry sky appearance.

17. Reed-Sternberg giant cell is a histological feature of:

A. Non-Hodgkin's lymphoma
B. Hodgkin's lymphoma
C. Burkitt's lymphoma
D. Ewing's sarcoma

Ans: (B)

18. **"Cart wheel or Checkerboard" pattern is a histological feature of:**

A. Ewing's sarcoma B. Multiple myeloma
C. Burkitt's lymphoma D. Kaposi's sarcoma

Ans: (B) Eccentrically placed nuclei with chromatin clumping round cells gives this appearance.

19. **Following types are histological type of osteosarcoma, *except:***

A. Osteoblastic B. Chondroblastic
C. Fibroblastic D. Periosteal osteosarcoma

Ans: (D) Periosteal osteosarcoma is clinical type not a histological type.

20. **In HIV infected patient most commonest vascular lesion is:**

A. Hemangioma B. Ewing's sarcoma
C. Kaposi's sarcoma D. Hemangioendothelioma

Ans: (C)

21. **"Stag horn" pattern of vascular slit is seen in:**

A. Hemangioma B. Hemangiopericytoma
C. Hemangioendothelioma D. Kaposi's sarcoma

Ans: (B)

22. **It's an example of hamartoma:**

A. Hemangioma B. Hemangioendothelioma
C. Hemangiopericytoma D. Kaposi's sarcoma

Ans: (A) Abnormal proliferation of tissues of structures native to the part is called hamartoma.

23. **African jaw lymphoma exclusively occurs in:**

A. Newborns B. Adults
C. Old age D. Children

Ans: (D) Age between 2 to 14 years.

24. Benign smooth mucle tumor is called:

A. Rhabdomyoma
B. Angiomyoma
C. Leiomyoma
D. Granular cell myoblastoma

Ans: (C)

25. Rhabdomyosarcoma is:

A. Malignant skeletal muscle lesion
B. Benign skeletal muscle tumor
C. Benign smooth muscle tumor
D. Both A and B

Ans: (A)

26. "Racquet", "Strap", Ribbon" cells with eosinophilic cytoplasm is a feature of:

A. Granular cell myoblastoma
B. Rhabdomyosarcoma
C. Leiomyosarcoma
D. Angiomyoma

Ans: (B)

27. Multiple neurofibroma, "Café au lait" spots and endocrine disturbances are the features of:

A. von Recklinghausen's disease
B. Neurilemmoma
C. Neurofibrosarcoma
D. Melanotic ameloblastoma

Ans: (A)

28. Which primary carcinoma commonly metastasis to jaws:

A. Thyroid
B. Prostate
C. Breast
D. Lung

Ans: (C)

29. Antony type A and B, verocay bodies are H/P feature of:

A. Schwannoma
B. Neurofibroma
C. MEN syndrome
D. Traumatic neuroma

Ans: (A) Schwann's cells arranged parralel to each is called antony type A. Irregular arrangement with Verocay bodies is type B.

30. Presence of Bence Jones protein in urine is a hallmark of :

A. Multiple myeloma
B. Ewing's tumor
C. Plasmocytoma
D. Rhabdomyosarcoma

Ans: (A) This is an unusual protein which coagulates when the urine is heated to 40 to 60°C. and gets disappears when urine is boiled. It's seen in 60 to 85 percentage of myeloma patient.

31. Onion skin appearance is the radiographic feature of:

A. Kaposi's sarcoma
B. Ewing's sarcoma
C. Multiple myeloma
D. Plasmcytoma

Ans: (B) New subperiosteal bone formation gives onion skin appearance in X–ray.

8

Healing of Oral Wounds

1. **Following factors favor wound healing, *except:***
   A. Hyperthermia B. Healthy vascular circulation
   C. Dehydration D. Normal diet

   Ans: (C) Dehydration delays wound healing.

2. **Removal of tissue from the living organism for the diagnostic study is called:**
   A. Autopsy B. Biopsy
   C. Cytology D. All of the above

   Ans: (B)

3. **Commonly used fixative in routine H/P laboratory is:**
   A. 10% alcohol B. 10% formalin
   C. 90 % formalin D. 90% alcohol

   Ans: (B)

4. **A small piece of tissue removed from the large lesion and subjected for histopathological study known as:**
   A. Incisional biopsy B. Excisional biopsy
   C. Exfoliative biopsy D. All of the above

   Ans: (A)

5. **Following statements are true regarding healing by secondary intention, *except:***
   A. Wound is filled with granulation tissue
   B. Edges cannot be approximated
   C. Wound contraction is significant
   D. Close approximation of the edges of the wound

   Ans: (D) This is true for healing by primary intention.

6. **Exfoliative cytology is more useful in:**

A. Oral cancer
B. Cervical cancer
C. Thyroid tumor
D. Salivary gland tumor

Ans: (B)

7. **After the difficult or traumatic extraction, dislodgement of blood clot, foul odour, severe pain, the condition known as:**

A. Pulpitis
B. Alveolar osteitis
C. Osteomyelitis
D. Dentoalveolar abscess

Ans: (B)

8. **Following statements are complication of fracture healing, *except:***

A. Malunion
B. Nonunion
C. Callus formation
D. Fibrous union

Ans: (C) It is a process of healing.

9. **Insertion of vital or non-vital tooth into the same alveolar socket which it's avulsed is known as:**

A. Implantation
B. Transplantation
C. Avulsion
D. Reimplantation

Ans: (D)

10. **Best media to carry the avulsed tooth is:**

A. Human blood
B. Patient's own saliva
C. Saline
D. Milk

Ans: (B)

9

Oral Aspects of Metabolic Disease

1. Normal serum calcium level of the body is about:

A. 9 to 11mg/dl B. 800 mg
C. 9 to 11 gm/dl D. 5 to 10 gm/dl

Ans: (A)

2. Following phenomenon are taking place due to low serum calcium level, *except:*

A. Stimulation of parathyroid hormone
B. Corpopedal spasm
C. Inhibition of parathyroid hormone
D. Hyperplasia or hypertrophy of parathyroid gland

Ans: (C)

3. Following factors retard absorption of calcium *except:*

A. Phytic acid B. Oxalic acid
C. Lactose D. Hypochlorhydria

Ans: (C)

4. Phosphate is absorbed by the intestine in the form of:

A. Orthophosphate B. Phosphoric acid
C. Phosphatase D. All of the above

Ans: (A)

5. Calcium deposition in the dead or degenerated tissues are known as:

A. Metastatic calcification B. Dystrophic calcification
C. Calcinosis cutis D. Hyalinization

Ans : (B)

6. **The term calcinosis denotes:**
   A. Deposition of calcium in the dead tissue
   B. Deposition of calcium in the living tissues
   C. Deposition of calcium in the hyalinized pulp
   D. Deposition of calcium in the skin

   Ans: (D)

7. **Following substances help for tubular reabsorption of sodium *except*:**
   A. Adrenalin B. Cortisone
   C. Desoxycortisone D. Hydrocortisone

   Ans: (A) It has a very negligible role in tubular reabsorption.

8. **Excretion of red colored urine, vesicle or bullous formation in the face and hands, red or brownish discoloration of deciduous and permanent teeth are feature of:**
   A. Mucopolysaccharidosis
   B. Amyloidosis
   C. Erythropoietic uroporphyria
   D. Hurler's syndrome

   Ans: (C) Congenital porphyia, inborn error in porphyrin metabolism.

9. **"Gargoyle cells" are seen in histopathology of:**
   A. Lipoid proteinosis B. Mucopolysaccharidosis
   C. Fructose intolerance D. Eosinophilic granuloma

   Ans: (B) Large metachromatic stained cells, finely granular with cresent shaped nucli, stained well in toulidine blue.

10. **Presence of nauseation, or vomiting sensation after taking fruits are clinical feature of:**
    A. Fructose intolerance B. Sucrose intolerance
    C. Lipoid proteinosis D. None of the above

    Ans: (A) It is due to hereditary deficiency of fructose 1-phosphate aldolase enzyme.

11. Non-lipid reticuloendothelial diseases are follows, *except:*

A. Hand-Schüller-Christian disease
B. Niemann- Pick disease
C. Letterer- Siwe Disease
D. Eosinophilic granuloma

Ans: (B) It is a lipid endotheliosis.

12. Kerasin deposition throughout the the reticuloendothelial system, presence of Gaucher's cell are the features of:

A. Eosinophilic granuloma
B. Niemann- Pick disease
C. Gaucher's disease
D. Eosinophilic granuloma

Ans: (C) These are round pale cell, eccentric nuclei, wrinkled or " crumpled silk" cytoplasm, measuring about 20 to 80 microns.

13. "Punched-out"bone destruction in one or multiple bones, exophthalmos. Diabetes insipidus is a traid, seen in:

A. Multifocal eosinophilic granuloma
B. Unifocal eosinophilic granuloma
C. Letterer–Siwe disease.
D. Histiocytosis X disease

Ans: (A) Also called as Hand-Schüller-Christian disease involves both skeletal and extra-skeletal system.

14. In which vitamin deficiency lack of histo-and morpho-differentiation occurs in the odontogenic epithelium cells:

A. Vitamin C
B. Vitamin B
C. Vitamin A
D. Vitamin D

Ans: (C)

15. The vitamin which has a substantial role in calcium and phosphorus homeostasis is:

A. Vitamin C
B. Vitamin B
C. Vitamin A
D. Vitamin D

Ans: (D) It activates the calcium binding protein.

16. Following statements are true regarding osteomalacia *except:*

A. It's also called adult's rickets
B. Flat bones and diaphyses of the long bones are affected
C. Males are affected by this disease
D. Postmenopausal females are commonly affected

Ans: (C)

17. "Scorbutic lattice" formed in the metaphysis of the bones. It's due to deficiency of:

A. Vitamin C B. Vitamin A
C. Vitamin B D. Vitamin D

Ans: (A) In scurvey failure of osteoblast to form osteoid matrix over the calcified cartilage, results zone of calcified but non-ossified matrix, named scorbutic lattice.

18. Engorged, mushroom shaped fungiform papillae and atrophic filiform papillae are the characteristic features of:

A. Thiamin deficiency B. Vitamin B_6 deficiency
C. Ariboflavinosis D. B_1 deficiency

Ans: (C)

19. Pellagra is due to:

A. Pyridoxine deficiency B. Niacin deficiency
C. Riboflavin deficiency D. Thiamin

Ans: (B)

20. Following statements regarding "Gigantism" are true, *except:*

A. Hyperpituitaric condition
B. Increase in number of acidophilic cells in anterior pituitary
C. It occurs before completion the epiphyseal growth
D. It occurs after the epiphyseal growth

Ans: (D) After the epiphyseal growth is called acromegaly.

21. **Brown's tumor is a feature of:**
   A. Hyperthyroidism
   B. Hypopituitarism
   C. Secondary hyperparathyroidism
   D. Primary hyperparathyroidism

   Ans: (C)

22. **A giant cell tumor is a feature of:**
   A. Primary hyperparathyroidism
   B. Secondary hyperparathyroidism
   C. Hyperthyroidism
   D. Hypoparathyroidism

   Ans: (A)

23. **Bronzing of the skin, brown pigmentation of the mucous membrane, vomiting, diarrhea and anemia are feature of:**
   A. Hyperfunction of the adrenal gland
   B. Addison's disease
   C. Diabetes mellitus
   D. Progeria

   Ans: (B)

24. **Dry mouth is a feature of altered secretion of which hormone:**
   A. Adrenalin
   B. Thyroxin
   C. Insulin
   D. Pituitary

   Ans: (C) Lack of insulin secretion in diabetic mellitus patient c/o dryness of the mouth.

25. **Cushing's syndrome is due to hyperfunction:**
   A. Thyroid gland
   B. Parathyroid gland
   C. Islet of pancreas
   D. Adrenal gland

   Ans: (D) Also occurs in increased secretion of ACTH.

10

Diseases of the Blood and Blood Forming Organ

1. The term Poikilocytosis denotes:

A. Variation in the size of the cell
B. Variation in the shape of the cell
C. Change in the nuclear shape of the cell
D. All of the above

Ans: (B) Variation in the size of the cell is called anisocytosis.

2. The main culprit to cause pernicious anemia is due to deficiency of:

A. Vitamin B_{12} B. Vitamin B_6
C. Vitamin C D. Gastric mucosal atrophy

Ans: (A) Also called as extrinsic factor for pernicious anemia.

3. The glossitis found in pernicious anemia is named as:

A. Bald tongue of sandwith
B. Moeller's glossitis
C. Migratory glossitis
D. Non-specific glossitis

Ans (B) Otherwise called Hunter's glossitis.

4. The term "Steatorrhea" denotes:

A. Excessive amount of calcium passing through the stools
B. Excessive amount of fat passing in the urine
C. Excess of fat pass through the stools
D. Both fat and calcium pass through the stools

Ans: (C) This condition commonly occurs in "Sprue" "Celiac disease".

5. The congenital aplastic anemia associated with syndrome is called:

A. Cooley's anemia
B. Sickle cell syndrome
C. Gray baby syndrome
D. Fanconi's syndrome

Ans: (D) Also associated with bone abnormalities, microcephaly, hypogenitalism olive – brown pigmentation of the skin.

6. Pathogenesis of thalassemia is:

A. Reduced in hemoglobin concentration
B. Defect in hemoglobin synthesis
C. Decrease in RBC count
D. All of the above

Ans: (B) Diminished synthesis of alpha and beta chain of hemoglobin A.

7. "Hair on end" appearance in radiographic feature of the skull seen in:

A. Thalassemia
B. Sickle cell anemia
C. Erythroblastosis fetalis
D. Leukemia

Ans: (A) Due to abnormal thickening of diploe, in between trabeculae become elongated, producing bristle like "crew cut" or "hair on end" appearance. Also seen in sickle cell anemia.

8. The type of hemoglobin formed in sickle cell anemia is:

A. HbA   B. HbB
C. HbS   D. HbM

Ans: (C) Normal adult (HbA) is genetically altered to produce sickle hemoglobin (HbS) by the substitution of valine for glutamine in the 6th position of the beta globin chain.

9. **Intrinsic stain in the dentition, ground section of these teeth give positive test for bilirubin, the condition is known as:**
   A. Hemosiderosis
   B. Chromogenic bacterial stains
   C. Tetracycline stains
   D. Erythroblastosis fetalis

   Ans: (D) It produces green, brown, or blue hue involving enamel extend into dentin in the developing tooth.

10. **Plummer-Vinson syndrome is a:**
   A. Premalignant lesion B. Premalignant condition
   C. Malignant lesion D. None of the above

   Ans: (B) Symptom complex of iron deficiency anemia, postcricoid web, koilonychia, progressive atrophy of the mucosa prone for malignant transformation.

11. **Abnormal increase in the number of RBCs in the peripheral blood, is defined as:**
   A. Polycythemia B. Leukemia
   C. Thrombocytosis D. Leukopenia

   Ans: (A)

12. **Epstein-Barr virus causes following diseases *except:***
   A. Infectious mononucleosis
   B. Chèdiak-Higashi syndrome
   C. Burkitt's lymphoma
   D. Nasopharyngeal carcinoma

   Ans: (B)

13. **The following disease is called as ' Kissing disease':**
   A. Glandular fever B. Cyclic neutropenia
   C. Burkitt's lymphoma D. Polycythemia vera

   Ans: (A) Also called as infectious mononucleosis.

14. Paul-Bunnell test is positive in:

A. Cyclic neutropenia
B. Agranulocytosis
C. Leukemia
D. Infectious mononucleosis

Ans (D)

15. Hemophilia A is due to:

A. Deficiency of antihemophilic globulin
B. Deficiency of plasma thromboplastin component
C. Deficiency of plasma thromboplastin antectent
D. von Willebrand's factor

Ans: (A)

11

Diseases of the Periodontium

1. Following statements regarding pellicle are true *except:*

A. It is formed immediately after the brushing
B. Completely covers the tooth surface
C. Mature thickness is about 0.1 to 0.8 microns
D. It is filled with bacteria

Ans: (D) It is mucoprotein or glycoprotein, free from bacteria.

2. All given stains in the teeth are produced by exogenous substances, *except:*

A. Tobacco tar B. Tetracycline
C. Chlorhexidine mouth wash D. Chromogenic bacteria

Ans (B) It is endogenous stain due to administration of tetracycline during formative stage of tooth.

3. Causative organism for ANUG is:

A. Borrelia vincenti B. Fusiform bacilli
C. Spirochetes D. Both A and B

Ans: (D) It is a fusospirochetal infection.

4. Drugs most commonly cause gingival enlargement are:

A. Antihypertensive B. Antiepileptic
C. Both A and B D. Only B

Ans: (C) Both these drugs calcium channel blocker in anti-hypertensive drug also causes gingival enlargement.

5. Following systemic factors causing gingival enlargement *except:*

A. Vitamin C deficiency B. Pregnancy
C. Leukemia D. Poor oral hygiene

Ans: (D) It is a local factor causing gingival enlargement.

6. The term gingival recession denotes:

A. Gingiva enlarges and covers the CE junction.
B. Gingiva moves towards apex exposes the cementum
C. Gingival covers the whole tooth
D. None of the above

Ans: (B)

7. Periodontal pocket extends apical to the crest of the alveolar bone is called:

A. Infrabony pocket B. Suprabony pocket
C. Pseudo pocket D. All of the above

Ans: (A)

8. If the pathological changes limited to the gingiva, gingival tissue increases in bulk that increases probing depth is called:

A. Infrabony pocket B. Suprabony pocket
C. Pseudo pocket D. Four walled pocket

Ans: (C)

9. Periodontosis is otherwise called:

A. Juvenile periodontitis
B. Desquamative gingivitis
C. Rapidly progressive periodontitis
D. Periodontal traumatism

Ans: (A)

10. Juvenile periodontosis, with Palmar-Plantar hyper-keratosis, calcification of Falx cerebri are feature of:

A. Papillon-Lefevre syndrome
B. Gardner's syndrome
C. Melkeron-Rosenthal syndrome
D. Hereditary ectodermal dysplasia

Ans: (A)

12

Physical and Chemical Injuries of the Oral Cavity

1. Habitual grinding of the teeth during sleep is called:

A. Traumatism B. Bruxism
C. Odontonomy D. Occlusal grinding

Ans: (B) This habit is commonly performed either during sleep or unconsciously during other activities.

2. Following statements are effect of bruxism on periodontium *except:*

A. Gingival recession B. Masticatory muscle spasm
C. Drifting of tooth D. Alveolar bone loss

Ans: (B) Effect of bruxism on muscles.

3. Ranula is a:

A. Mucocele in the anterior lingual salivary gland duct
B. Mucocele in the parotid duct
C. Mucocele in the sublingual gland duct
D. Mucocele in the submandibular duct

Ans: (C) Occurs in the floor of the mouth.

4. Commonest site for sialolithiasis is:

A. Minor salivary gland ducts B. Parotid ducts
C. Sublingual duct D. Submandibular duct

Ans: (D) Tortuous course of duct and thick mucous secretion are cause for sialolithiasis in submandibular duct.

5. Plumbism is due to:

A. Mercury poisoning B. Lead poisoning
C. Bismuth poisoning D. Arsenic poisoning

Ans: (B)

6. **Grayish line or bluish black line in gingiva, excessive salivation, metallic taste, salivary gland swelling are features of:**

A. Lead poisoning B. Bismuth poisoning
C. Mercury poisoning D. Arsenic poisoning

Ans : (A) Also systemically peripheral neuritis, causes wrist drop or foot drop.

7. **Following features are due to mercurial poisoning *except:***

A. Pink discoloration of skin and mucous membrane
B. Pink tooth
C. Drippling of saliva
D. Gastrointestinal diturbances

Ans: (B) Pink tooth occurs due to internal resorption of the tooth.

8. **Intensity of browish discoloration of tooth caused by which of the following tetracycline:**

A. Chlortetracycline B. Oxytetracycline
C. Doxycycline D. All of the above

Ans: (A)

9. **Allergic reaction in the skin or mucous membrane after repeated contact of causative agent is known as:**

A. Drug allergy B. Idiosynergetic reaction
C. Stomatitis venenata D. Drug sensitivity

Ans: (C)

10. **Smooth diffuse edematous swelling around the lips, chin, eyes and the tongue after administration of chemical substances is known as:**

A. Drug sensitivity
B. Contact stomatitis
C. Stomatitis medicamentosa
D. Angioneurotic edema

Ans: (D)

13

Diseases of Skin

1. Hypohidrosis, hypotrichosis, hypodontia are features of:

A. Hereditary hypohidrotic ectodermal dysplasia
B. Hereditary benign intraepithelial dyskeratosis
C. Chondroectodermal dysplasia
D. Ectodermal dysplasia

Ans: (A)

2. Ellis-van Creveld syndrome is associated with:

A. Chondroectodermal dysplasia
B. Hereditary hypohidrotic ectodermal dysplasia
C. Lichen planus
D. Pemphigus

Ans: (A)

3. Lichen planus has prominent clinical feature of:

A. Nikolsky's sign B. Auspitz's sign
C. Wickham's striae D. All of the above

Ans: (C)

4. Grinspan's syndrome is associated with:

A. Lichen planus B. Psoriasis
C. Pemphigus foliaceous D. Erythema multiforme

Ans: (A)

5. Hypertension, Diabetes mellitus, lichen planus:

A. Grinspan's syndrome B. Stevens-Johnson syndrome
C. Gardner's syndrome D. Kawasaki syndrome

Ans: (A)

6. Following are types of lichen planus *except:*

A. Reticular B. Erosive
C. Atrophic D. Ulcerative

Ans: (D)

7. Saw tooth retepegs is a histological feature of:

A. Lichen planus B. Psoriasis
C. Pemphigus D. Erythema multiforme

Ans: (A)

8. Most common dermatological disease is:

A. Lichen planus B. Psoriasis
C. Erythema multiforme D. White sponge nevus

Ans: (B)

9. Tiny bleeding spot after removal of deep scales shown in psoriasis is known as:

A. Nikolsky's sign B. Wickham's straie
C. Auspitz's sign D. Tzank test

Ans: (C)

10. IgG and IgA serum levels in psoriasis:

A. Decreased B. Increased
C. Average D. No change

Ans: (B)

11. Psoriasiform lesions of oral mucosa associated with:

A. Reiter's syndrome
B. Benign migratory glossitis
C. Ectopic geographic tongue
D. All of the above

Ans: (D)

12. Primary lesion or Herald spot is shown in:

A. Psoriasis B. Pityriasis rosea
C. Erythema multiforme D. Lichen planus

Ans: (D)

13. Erythema multiforme associated with:

A. Grinspan syndrome
B. Darier's disease
C. Stevens-Johnson syndrome
D. Plummer-Vinson syndrome

Ans: (C)

14. "Target" lesion or Bull's eye lesions are the features of:

A. Psoriasis B. Erythema multiforme
C. Lichen planus D. Pemphigus

Ans: (B)

15. Stevens-Johnson syndrome is severe—form of erythema multiforme.

A. Papule B. Macule
C. Pustul D. Bullous

Ans: (D)

16. In Stevens-Johnson syndrome lesion focused in:

A. Skin B. Eye
C. Oral cavity D. All of the above

Ans: (D)

17. Mucocutaneous lymph node syndrome:

A. Darier's disease B. Kawasaki disease
C. Cannon's disease D. Tzank's disease

Ans: (A)

18. Kearatosis follicuris is:

A. Darier's disease B. Kawasaki's disease
C. Cannon's disease D. Tzanck's disease

Ans: (A)

19. Cannon's diseases is associated with:

A. Lichen planus B. Candidiasis
C. White sponge nevus D. Dyskeratosis congenita

Ans: (C)

20. Pemphigus has following type *except:*

A. Pemphigus vulgaris B. Pemphigus bullous
C. Pemphigus vegetans D. Pemphigus foliaceus

Ans: (B)

21. Nikolsky's sign is shown in:

A. Pemphigus vegetans B. Pemphigus foliaceus
C. Pemphigus erythematosus D. Pemphigus vulgaris

Ans: (D)

22. Nikolsky's sign is characterized by:

A. Perivascular edema B. Perivasicular edema
C. Prevesicular edema D. Prevascular edema

Ans: (C)

23. Brazilian pemphigus is an endemic form of:

A. Pemphigus vulgaris B. Pemphigus vegetans
C. Pemphigus foliaceus D. Pemphigus erythematosus

Ans: (C)

24. Snear usher syndrome is associated with:

A. Pemphigus vulgaris B. Pemphigus vegetans
C. Pemphigus foliaceus D. Pemphigus erythematosus

Ans: (D)

25. One of the classical histological feature of pemphigus vulgaris is:

A. Suprabasilar split B. Subbasilar split
C. Perivascular edema D. None of the above

Ans: (A)

26. Tzanck's cells are present in:

A. Pemphigus B. Erythema multiforme
C. Lichen planus D. Psoriasis

Ans: (A)

27. Most common immunoglobulin found in pemphigus are:

A. IgA
B. IgG
C. IgM
D. C3 with IgA and IgM

Ans: (A)

28. Hailey-Hailey disease is also called as:

A. Cicatricial pemphigoid
B. Familial benign chronic pemphigus
C. Bullous pemphigoid
D. Pemphigus vulgaris

Ans: (B)

29. Benign mucous membrane pemphigoid is also known as:

A. Familial benign chronic pemphigus
B. Bullous pemphigoid
C. Cicatricial pemphigoid
D. Pemphigus

Ans: (C)

30. Parapemphigus is:

A. Bullous pemphigoid
B. Cicatricial pemphigoid
C. Familial benign chronic pemphigus
D. None of the above

Ans: (A)

31. Butterfly shaped lesion is seen in:

A. Discoid lupus erythematosus
B. Systemic lupus erythematosus
C. Both A and B
D. Erythema multiforme

Ans: (C)

32. "Carpet tack" extension of lesions are shown in:

A. Systemic lupus erythematosus
B. Erythema multiforme
C. Lichen planus
D. Discoid lupus erythematosus

Ans: (D)

33. Crest syndrome is associated with:

A. Erythema multiforme B. Systemic sclerosis
C. Psoriasis D. Pemphigus

Ans: (B)

34. Cutis hyperelastica is associated with:

A. Ehlers-Danlos syndrome B. Erythema multiforme
C. Systemic sclerosis D. None of the above

Ans: (A)

35. Goltz-Gorlin syndrome is associated with:

A. Focal dermal hypoplasia syndrome
B. Solar elastosis
C. Ehlers-Danlos syndrome
D. All of the above

Ans: (A)

36. Mask like appearance of the face and claw like appearance of hands is seen in:

A. Ehlers–Danlos syndrome B. Systemic sclerosis
C. Focal dermal hypoplasia D. None of the above

Ans: (B)

37. Two chief forms of systemic sclerosis:

A. Diffuse systemic B. Localized
C. Morphea type D. Both A and C

Ans: (D)

38. Following are types of epidermolysis bullosa, *except:*

A. Epidermolysis bullosa simplex
B. Epidermolysis bullosa dystrophic
C. Epidermolysis bullosa acquired
D. Epidermolysis bullosa hypertrophic

Ans: (D)

39. Nikolsky' s sign is seen in:

A. Pemphigus vulgaris
B. Familial benign chronic pemphigus
C. Epidermolysis bullosa
D. Both A and B

Ans: (D)

40. Test usually performed in pemphigus

A. Paul-Bunnel test
B. Immunofluorescent test
C. Dark field microscope
D. Tzanck test

Ans: (D)

41. Dyskeratosis congenita is a disease involving:

A. Bone
B. Genitalia
C. Skin
D. Eyes

Ans: (C)

42. Isolated Darier's disease is:

A. Warty dyskeratoma
B. Incontinentia pigment
C. Dyskeratosis congenita
D. None of the above

Ans: (A)

43. Bloch - Sulzberger syndrome is associated with:

A. Warty dyskeratoma
B. Incontinentia pigment
C. Dyskeratosis congenita
D. None of the above

Ans: (B)

44. Suprabasilar split is histopathological feature of:

A. Lichen planus
B. Pemphigus vulgaris
C. Pemphigus foliaceus
D. Erythema multiforme

Ans: (B)

45. Subepidermal vesicle seen in:

A. Erythema multiforme
B. Pemphigus
C. Lichen planus
D. Epidermolysis bullosa

Ans: (A)

46. Eye lesion seen in Stevens-Johnson syndromes are:

A. Photophobia
B. Keratocongunctivitis sicca
C. Corneal ulceration
D. All of the above

Ans: (D)

47. Drugs that trigger erythema multiforme, *except:*

A. Phenylbutazone
B. Barbiturates
C. Paracetamol
D. Sulfonamides

Ans: (C)

48. Ectodermosis erosive pluriorificialis is the other name of:

A. Ectodermal bullosa
B. Ectodermal dysplasia
C. Erythema multiforme
D. Systemic lupus erythematosus

Ans: (C)

49. Hereditary hypohidrotic ectodermal dysplasia is a:

A. X-linked dominant character
B. X-linked recessive character
C. Autosomal resseive character
D. None of the above

Ans: (A)

50. Congenital ectodermal defect is applied to:

A. Erythema multiforme
B. Hereditary hypohidrotic ectodermal dysplasia
C. Lichen planus
D. Psoriasis

Ans: (B)

14

Diseases of Bone and Joints

1. **'Brittle Bone Disease" is the other name of:**
   - A. Osteopetrosis
   - B. Osteogenesis imperfecta
   - C. Osteitis deformans
   - D. Fibrous dysplasia

   Ans: (B) Bones increases porosity fragility, prone for fracture.

2. **Pale blue sclera is a prominent sign in the following diseases, *except:***
   - A. Normal infants
   - B. Fetal rickets
   - C. Down's syndrome
   - D. Marfan's syndrome

   Ans: (C) Due to thin sclera choroid colour reflects through it.

3. **Infantile cortical hyperostosis is also known as:**
   - A. Caffey's disease
   - B. Marie and Sainton's disease
   - C. Crouzon disease
   - D. Treacher Collins syndrome

   Ans: (A)

4. **Gross thickening and sclerosis of the cortex is the classical roentgenographic feature of:**
   - A. Infantile cortical hyperostosis
   - B. Mandibulofacial dysostosis
   - C. Craniofacial dysostosis
   - D. Achondroplasia

   Ans: (A)

5. The common feature of both cleidocranial dysplasia and Gardner's syndrome is:

A. Early loss of deciduous teeth

B. Prolonged retention of deciduous teeth and multiple supernumerary teeth

C. Multiple impacted permanent teeth

D. Intestinal polyposis

Ans: (B)

6. Absence of cellular cementum is seen in:

A. Caffey's disease B. Craniofacial dysostosis

C. Cleidocranial dysplasia D. Crouzon's disease

Ans: (C) Absence or paucity of the cellular cementum in both permanent and deciduous teeth.

7. Crouzon's disease is also called as:

A. Mandibulofacial dysostosis

B. Osteopetrosis

C. Craniofacial dysostosis

D. Osteitis deformens

Ans: (C)

8. Unusual mobility of the shoulders, defects of vertebral column and bones of the digits are the feature of:

A. Achondroplasia

B. Pierre Robin syndrome

C. Cleidocranial dysplasia

D. Osteitis deformens

Ans: (C)

9. Craniosynostotic syndrome occurring with syndactyly is:

A. Down's syndrome B. Marfan's syndrome

C. Apert's syndrome D. Cherubism

Ans: (C)

10. Craniofacial dysostosis has followig feature *except:*

A. Triangular frontal defect
B. Hypertelorism
C. Exophthalmous
D. Blind fistula

Ans: (D)

11. Syndrome associated with mandibulofacial dysostosis, *except:*

A. Treacher Collins syndrome
B. Marfan's syndrome
C. Brancheal arch syndrome
D. Franceschetti's syndrome

Ans: (B) Marfan's syndrome associated with collagen disorder.

12. Retardation or failure of differentiation of maxillary mesoderm resuls in:

A. Mandibulofacial dysostosis
B. Craniofacial dysostosis
C. Cleidocranial dysplasia
D. Marfan's syndrome

Ans: (A)

13. Characteristic 'Bird face' is a feature of:

A. Down syndrome
B. Marfan syndrome
C. Pierre Robin syndrome
D. Mandibulofacial dysostosis

Ans: (D) Arrested development of mandible resulted in 'bird facies'.

14. Long thin extremities and arachnodactyly is a clinical feature of:

A. Marfan's syndrome
B. Down's syndrome
C. Robin anamalad
D. None of the above

Ans: (A) Excessive length of tubular bone occurs in Marfan's syndrome.

15. In Down's syndrome cytogenetic investigation reveals chromosomal aberration in:

A. Chromosome 23 B. Chromosome 27
C. Chromosome 47 D. Chromosome 21

Ans: (D)

16. In Down's syndrome, which form of genetic disorder commonly found:

A. Trisomy 21
B. Translocation
C. Chromosomal mosaicism
D. All are equally distributed

Ans: (A) About 95% are trisomy 21 with 47 chromosomes.

17. Normal bone apposition, but failure of bone resorption is characteristic feature of:

A. Osteopetrosis B. Down's syndrome
C. Osteitis deformens D. Fibrous dysplasia

Ans: (A) Deficient osteoclastic activity, parathormone activity.

18. RBC count is below 1 000,000 / cumm, increased acid phosphatase are the laboratory findings of:

A. Marble bone disease B. Achondroplasia
C. Robin anomalad D. Marfan's syndrome

Ans: (A) In benign dominant osteopetrosis.

19. Following are other name for osteopetrosis, *except*:

A. Marble bone disease B. Albers- Schönberg disease
C. Osteosclerosis D. Crouzon's disease

Ans: (D) Craniofacial dysostosis also called Crouzon disease.

20. Achondroplasia is a:

A. Disturbance in endochondral bone formation
B. Disturbance in intramembranous bone formation
C. Both A and B
D. Defect in hormanal metabolism

Ans: (A)

21. Marfan's syndrome is a hereditary disease transmitted by:

A. Autosomal recessive trait
B. Autosomal dominant trait
C. X-linked recessive trait
D. None of the above

Ans: (A)

22. Marfan's syndrome there is defective formation of:

A. Collagen
B. Osteoid matrix
C. Ground substances
D. Chondroid

Ans: (A)

23. Clinical feature of Marfan's syndrome *except:*

A. Dolichostenomelia
B. Arachodactyly
C. Kyphosis and scoliosis
D. Osteopetrosis

Ans: (D)

24. Severe form of osteopetrosis:

A. Malignant dominant osteopetrosis
B. Benign dominant osteopetrosis
C. Benign recessive osteopetrosis
D. Malignant recessive osteopetrosis

Ans: (D)

25. Skull form of achondroplasia:

A. Dolicocephalic skull
B. Mesocephalic skull
C. Brachycephalic skull
D. Normocephalic skull

Ans: (C)

26. Bone disorder caused by slow virus is:

A. Osteitis deformans
B. Acute sclerosing pancephalitis
C. Osteopetrosis
D. Both A and B

Ans: (D)

27. "Osteoporosis circumscripta" is an isolated lesion in the:

A. Skull
B. Femur
C. Clavicle
D. Sacrum

Ans: (A)

28. "Cotton wool" appearance in radiographic feature of:

A. Down's syndrome
B. Osteitis deformans
C. Marfan's syndrome
D. Fibrous dysplasia

Ans: (B)

29. Characteristic laboratory finding in Paget's disease is:

A. Increased serum calcium
B. Increased serum phosphate
C. Increased alkaline phosphatase
D. Increased acid phosphatase

Ans: (C)

30. "Mosaic bone" Jig saw–Puzzle appearance of bone are feature of:

A. Osteopetrosis
B. Osteitis deformans
C. Osteosarcoma
D. Sclerosing osteomyelitis

Ans: (B)

31. Differential diagnosis of Paget's disease *except:*

A. Fibrous dysplasia
B. Fibro-osteoma
C. Osteosarcoma
D. Osteolysis

Ans: (D)

32. Vanishing bone disease is the other name for:

A. Osteopetrosis
B. Osteitis deformans
C. Massive osteolysis
D. Osteosarcoma

Ans: (C)

33. Fibrous dysplasia is a fibro-osseous disease characterized by fibrous tissue replaced with:

A. Metaplastic bone formation
B. Malignant bone formation
C. Dysplastic bone formation
D. Normal bone formation

Ans: (A)

34. "Café au lait" spot is a feature of type of fibrous dysplasia:

A. Polyostotic fibrous dysplasia
B. Monostotic fibrous dysplasia
C. Both A and B
D. Cherubism

Ans: (A)

35. Fibrous dysplasia of multiple bones, pigmented lesion of the skin, and endocrine disturbance is shown in:

A. Jaffe's type
B. Albert's syndrome
C. Apert's syndrome
D. Albright's syndrome

Ans: (D)

36. Name craniofacial fibrous dysplasia usually given to fibrous dysplasia affecting:

A. Mandible
B. Maxilla
C. Zygomatic
D. All of the above

Ans: (B)

37. Ground–glass /peau d' orange is a radiological feature of:

A. Fibrous dysplasia
B. Cleidocranial dysplasia
C. Osteitis deformans
D. Marfan's syndrome

Ans: (A)

38. Typical histological feature of fibrous dysplasia:

A. "C" shaped trabeculae
B. Jig saw –puzzle appearance
C. Starry sky appearance
D. Cart and wheel appearance

Ans: (A)

39. Cherubism is:

A. Familial fibrous dysplasia of the jaws
B. Hereditary fibrous dysplasia of the jaws
C. Juvenile fibrous dysplasia
D. All of the above

Ans: (D)

40. Failure of development of condyle is termed:

A. Aplasia of the condyle
B. Hypoplasia of the condyle
C. Metaplasia of the condyle
D. Neoplasia of the condyle

Ans: (A)

41. Complete dislocation of TMJ:

A. Subluxation B. Luxation
C. Ankylosis D. All of the above

Ans: (B)

42. Hypomobility of TMJ is due to:

A. Luxation B. Subluxation
C. Ankylosis D. None of the above

Ans: (C)

43. Temporomandibular joint pain – dysfunction syndrome, masticatory myalgia syndrome are all associated with:

A. Ankylosis
B. Luxation
C. Subluxation
D. Myofacial pain dysfunction syndrome

Ans: (D)

44. Etiology of myofacial pain dysfunction syndrome is:

A. Ankylosis B. Luxation
C. Masticatory muscle spasm D. None of the above

Ans: (C)

45. Muscle spasm in MPDS is due to:

A. Muscular over contraction B. Muscular over extension
C. Muscle fatigue D. All of the above

Ans: (D)

46. The theory based on myofacial pain dysfunction syndrome:

A. Psychophysiologic theory B. Physiological theory
C. Sigmund-Freud theory D. Mechanical theory

Ans: (A)

47. Pain, muscle tenderness, clicking noise, limitation of jaw movement are all the clinical feature of:

A. Myofacial pain dysfunction syndrome
B. Myocardial infarction
C. Trigeminal neuralgia
D. Auriculotemporal neuralgia

Ans: (A)

48. Rheumatoid arthritis is common in:

A. Male B. Children
C. Elderly persons D. Female

Ans: (D)

49. Arthritis:

A. Inflammation of bone
B. Inflammation of joints
C. Inflammation of soft tissues
D. Inflammation of auricle

Ans: (B)

50. Fracture of the condyle shows:

A. Pain B. Swelling
C. Limitation of movement D. All of the above

Ans: (D)

51. **Arthritis due to infection is caused by:**
    A. Streptococci
    B. Staphylococci
    C. Pneumococci
    D. Anthrax

    Ans: (A)

52. **Rheumatoid arthritis in children in TMJ known as:**
    A. Still's disease
    B. Caffe's disease
    C. Robinson's disease
    D. Gene's disease

    Ans: (A)

53. **Degenerative joint disorder is known as:**
    A. Osteomyelitis
    B. Osteoarthritis
    C. Osteosarcoma
    D. Osteoid osteoma

    Ans: (B)

54. **Clicking and snapping of joints are features of:**
    A. Ankylosis
    B. Osteoarthritis
    C. Traumatic arthritis
    D. All of the above

    Ans: (B)

15

Tumors of Salivary Gland

1. **The etiology of Mikulicz's disease is:**

   A. Viral B. Bacterial
   C. Autoimmune D. Genetic

   Ans: (C)

2. **Most common salivary gland tumor is:**

   A. Basal cell adenoma B. Pleomorphic adenoma
   C. Canalicular adenoma D. Oxiphilic adenoma

   Ans: (B) Pleomorphic adenoma about 90% occurrence among salivary gland tumours.

3. **Warthin's tumor is also called:**

   A. Benign lymphoepithelial lesion
   B. Papillary cystadenoma lymphomatosam
   C. Canalicular adenoma
   D. Sialadenoma papilliferum

   Ans: (B) Papillary cystadenoma lymphomatosam, adeno-lymphoma.

4. **Radiographic feature shows branchless fruit laden tree, cherry blossom appearance seen in following condition:**

   A. Sjögren's syndrome B. Mikulicz's disease
   C. Warthin's tumor D. Cylindroma

   Ans: (A)

5. **Sialolith commonly occurs in:**

   A. Sublingual salivary gland B. Maxillary sinus
   C. Submandibular salivary gland D. Parotid gland

   Ans: (C) Due to thick mucus secretion, and tortuous course of duct.

6. A benign inflammatory disease of salivary gland which mimics both clinical and histological picture of malignancy is:

A. Benign lymphoepithelial lesion
B. Sjögren syndrome
C. Mikulicz's disease
D. Necrotizing sialometaplasia

Ans: (D) Necrotizing sialometaplasia.

7. Tumor cells arranged in cribriform pattern,swiss chesse pattern, and honeycomb arrangement, are characteristic feature of:

A. Acinic cell carcinoma
B. Mucoepidermoid carcinoma
C. Adenoid cystic carcinoma
D. Salivary duct carcinoma

Ans: (C) Adenoid cystic carcinoma or cylindroma.

8. Caries activity increased in following salivary gland diseased condition, known as:

A. Malignant disease of salivary gland
B. Xerostomia
C. Profuse salivation
D. Kimura's disease

Ans: (B) Dryness of the mouth or xerostomia.

9. Comedo type of necrosis seen in:

A. Salivary duct carcinoma
B. Cylindroma
C. Acinic cell carcinoma
D. Pleomorphic adenoma

Ans: (A) Necrosis around the salivary duct known as comedo necrosis.

10. Following laboratory investigation is positive in Sjögren's syndrome *except:*

A. Polyclonal hyperglobulinemia
B. Rheumatoid factor
C. Antinuclear antibodies
D. Bence Jones protein

Ans: (D) Positive in multiple myeloma.

11. "Epi-myoepithelial island" is the histopathological feature of:

A. Mikulicz's disease
B. Sjögren's syndrome
C. Kimura's disease
D. Ductal papilloma

Ans: (A) Proliferation of ductal and myoepithelial cells.

12. Perineural invasion is common feature found in:

A. Mucoepidermoid carcinoma
B. Clear cell carcinoma
C. Adenoid cystic carcinoma
D. Acinic cell carcinoma

Ans: (C) Spreads along perineural sheath or perineural space.

13. Mucus secreting cells, intermediate cells, epidermoid cells are seen in:

A. Epidermoid carcinoma
B. Mucoepidermoid carcinoma
C. Ductal carcinoma
D. Inverted duct papilloma

Ans: (B)

14. Most preferable site of occurrence for pleomorphic adenoma is:

A. Parotid gland
B. Submandibular gland
C. Blandin Nun
D. von Ebner gland

Ans: (A)

15. Following statements are true regarding histogenesis of central mucoepidermoid carcinoma, *except:*

A. Neoplastic transformation of entrapped retromolar mucous gland

B. Developmentally included embryonic remants of the submaxillary gland

C. Neoplastic transformation of the mucous secreting cells in dentigerous cyst

D. Neoplastic transformation of periapical cyst

Ans: (D)

16. "Party wall" arrangement of epithelial cells is a characteristic histologic feature of:

A. Canalicular adenoma

B. Basal cell adenoma

C. Warthin's tumor

D. Oncocytoma

Ans: (A) Long strands and cords of epithelial cells, arranged in a double row showing Party wall appearance.

READER SUGGESTIONS SHEET

Please help us to improve the quality of our publications by completing and returning this sheet to us.

Title/Author: **MCQs in Oral Pathology** *by K Karunakaran*

Your name and address:

Phone and Fax:

e-mail address:

How did you hear about this book? [please tick appropriate box (es)]

☐ Direct mail from publisher ☐ Conference ☐ Bookshop

☐ Book review ☐ Lecturer recommendation ☐ Friends

☐ Other (please specify) ☐ Website

Type of purchase: ☐ Direct purchase ☐ Bookshop ☐ Friends

Do you have any brief comments on the book?

Please return this sheet to the name and address given below.

JAYPEE BROTHERS
MEDICAL PUBLISHERS (P) LTD
EMCA House, 23/23B Ansari Road, Daryaganj
New Delhi 110 002, India